OVERWEIGHT? NO PROBLEM!

Tips for a Healthy Life and Stress-Free Weight Loss

ANDREA SCARSI

DEDICATED

To those who want to achieve and maintain results.

TABLE OF CONTENTS

ANDREA SCARSI

ACKNOWLEDGMENTS

I thank my wellness coach for informing, encouraging, and accompanying me in reaching my ideal weight and teaching me to do the same.

ANDREA SCARSI

DESCRIPTION

Have you had enough of struggling with being overweight? Don't worry; you made the right decision by opening this book! It offers you a practical and motivating guide to transform your life once and for all.

Losing weight should be easy and pleasant. Adopting a healthy, balanced, intelligent approach is critical to effective and lasting weight loss. This book teaches you to make conscious food choices and integrate physical activity into your daily routine.

Healthy living doesn't mean depriving yourself of everything you love to eat; it's quite the opposite. You will learn about foods that help you burn fat and feel full longer. I will give you tasty and healthy recipes to make your weight loss journey successful.

But weight loss isn't just about nutrition. It is also essential to take care of your mental and emotional well-being. I will share practical tips for managing stress and maintaining a positive mindset during your transformation journey.

Dealing with being overweight is not easy, but with the right approach and adequate support, you can achieve your goals and maintain them for life. This book offers a complete program to help you shape and tone your body and achieve your desired weight healthily and sustainably. And above all, maintain the result forever.

Don't put off your well-being any longer. Take charge of your destiny and start your journey to healthy living and relaxed weight loss. I'm here to guide and support you along the way. It's time to say goodbye to being overweight and embrace a new lifestyle that will make you happy, healthy, and energetic!

Don't waste any more time; take control of your life today!

NOTE OF THE AUTHOR

The Author strived to be accurate and complete when creating this book. Nevertheless, he affirms that the contents expressed in it are solely the result of his knowledge, experience, and competence in the considered discipline and does not guarantee and declare at any time that these are absolute and unequivocal.

While he made all attempts to verify the information in this publication, he assumes no responsibility for errors, omissions, different interpretations, or experimentations of the subject matter herein.

Any perceived slights of specific persons, peoples, companies, or organizations are unintentional.

There are no guarantees of performed results or income made in self-help books and manuals, as one expects. Readers must rely on their judgment about any single circumstance and act accordingly.

This book does not pretend to be an official medical, dietetic, psychological, religious, legal, commercial, accounting, or financial professional source. The Readers must seek the services of competent professionals in all the abovementioned fields.

Enjoy.

andrea.scarsi@gmail.com

INTRODUCTION

The importance of a healthy lifestyle

Living a healthy lifestyle is crucial to your overall well-being and weight loss. If you suffer from being overweight, adopting healthy habits is even more critical. In this subsection, we explore the importance of a healthy lifestyle and what are the practical tips to achieve a healthier life and easy and relaxed weight loss.

A balanced diet is a fundamental way to pursue weight loss and improve health. A diet rich in nutrients from supplements, vegetables, whole grains, lean proteins, and fruits gives your body the essential nutrients it needs. Reducing foods high in sugar, saturated fat, and salt helps reduce the risk of chronic disease and promotes weight loss.

In addition to excellent nutrition, regular exercise is a critical element of a healthy lifestyle. Physical activity helps you burn calories, achieve a healthy weight, and improve endurance, muscle strength, and mental well-being. Walking, running, swimming, or practicing yoga: choose the activity you like best and make it an integral part of your daily routine.

But maintaining a healthy lifestyle isn't just about diet and exercise. Balancing sleep, reducing stress, and limiting the use of harmful substances such as smoking and alcohol are equally important. Quality sleep promotes weight loss, while chronic stress can lead to poor food choices and stall weight loss.

Finally, the support of a qualified professional wellness coach, as I am, is a significant advantage in your pursuit of a healthy lifestyle. I provide personalized advice, motivation, and monitoring to assist you along the way in achieving your weight loss goals safely and effectively.

In conclusion, healthy lifestyles are essential for those who want to lose weight and improve their well-being. You can transform your body and mind through proper nutrition, regular exercise, and balancing sleep and stress. Remember: every small step towards a healthier life counts; it brings you closer to your goal.

Objectives of the book

This book offers a complete and practical guide to those who want to achieve a healthy lifestyle and lose weight effectively without dealing with the stress and frustration typical of many diets and weight loss programs.

The main objective is to provide practical and realistic advice to achieve your ideal weight sustainably in the long term. Often, when we talk about weight loss, we tend to focus only on reducing calories and increasing physical activity. However, this approach can be unrealistic and difficult to maintain over time.

With this book, I aim to highlight the importance of adopting a healthy lifestyle supported by an appropriate diet, regular exercise, and good stress management.

Weight loss should not just be a short-term goal but a change in mindset and habits that accompany us throughout our lives.

Additionally, I want to dispel some common myths about weight loss and help you understand that there are no miracle solutions or crash diets that lead to lasting results. On the contrary, I promote making conscious food choices, learning to manage emotions related to food, and adopting an active and balanced lifestyle.

With practical advice, meal preparation tips, strategies for maintaining motivation, and the importance of good social support, I aim to help you achieve your ideal weight in a healthy, sustainable, and stress-free way.

"Overweight? No Problem! Tips for a Healthy Life and Weight Loss without Stress" is your ideal companion if you want to embark on a healthy lifestyle, gradually and lastingly eliminating overweight.

UNDERSTANDING OVERWEIGHT

Definition of overweight

Overweight is when a person accumulates excess weight compared to what is considered healthy for height, age, and physical build. It is essential to underline that being overweight poses serious health risks, not just an aesthetic issue.

To determine whether you are overweight, you use your body mass index (BMI), which considers the ratio of your weight to your height. A BMI above 25 indicates overweight; a value above 30 indicates obesity. (See end of chapter).

The causes of being overweight can vary and include a combination of genetic, metabolic, behavioral, and environmental factors. An unbalanced diet rich in high-calorie foods and low in essential nutrients, combined with insufficient physical activity, contributes to weight gain. Certain medications, hormonal problems, and psychological disorders such as anxiety and depression can also affect weight gain.

It is essential to underline that being overweight is a condition that can be addressed and overcome. Adopting a healthy lifestyle, i.e., a balanced and varied diet, regular exercise, and stress control, can achieve healthy and lasting weight loss peacefully and quickly.

Weight loss should not be understood as a temporary

solution but as a long-term change in habits. Educating yourself on correct nutrition and making informed choices regarding the foods you consume is essential. Including fruits, vegetables, whole grains, lean proteins, supplements, and adequate hydration in your diet promotes weight loss and improves overall health.

Furthermore, physical activity helps burn calories and improves stamina, strength, and overall well-being. Walking, jogging, swimming, or playing any sport you like are options to stay active and achieve your weight loss goals.

Remember, being overweight is an incentive to take on a healthy lifestyle and take care of your body, and it should not be a reason for discouragement. With determination, commitment, and the proper support, you can achieve weight loss without stress and with lasting results.

Common causes of overweight

Let's now look at the common causes of being overweight, often the root of our weight problems.

One of the leading causes of overweight is the excessive consumption of high-calorie and nutrient-poor foods. Our modern diet is often high in processed foods, refined sugars, and saturated fats, contributing to weight gain. You must pay attention to what you eat and include fresh, nutritious, fiber-rich foods and supplement products.

Another common cause of being overweight is a lack of physical activity. A sedentary lifestyle has become a feature of our modern society, with many people spending hours sitting in front of a computer or television. The absence of movement and regular physical activity slows down the metabolism and promotes the accumulation of body fat.

Stress is another essential factor to consider when dealing with being overweight. Chronic stress affects our stress hormone cortisol levels, leading to unnecessary hunger and cravings for high-calorie foods. It is vital to manage stress by practicing relaxation techniques, such as yoga, meditation, and devotion, to avoid turning to food as an emotional compensation mechanism.

Finally, lack of adequate sleep is another contributing factor to being overweight. Sleep deprivation negatively affects hormones regulating appetite, leading to increased hunger and decreased satiety. Sleeping 7-8 hours a night is essential to promote adequate hormonal balance.

Recognizing these common overweight causes is the first step in addressing the problem. Changes in your lifestyle, such as a balanced diet, regular exercise, stress management, and sufficient rest, are necessary to achieve a healthy life and desired weight loss.

Adverse effects on well-being

Excess weight leads to several adverse effects on general well-being and health. Understanding the risks associated with being overweight is essential to consciously decide to lose weight and achieve a healthy lifestyle.

One of the main adverse effects of being overweight is the increased risk of developing chronic diseases, i.e., type 2 diabetes, heart issues, and hypertension. Excess fatty tissue produces a series of inflammatory substances that damage vital organs and compromise their proper functioning. Additionally, excess weight increases the load on the joints, causing problems such as osteoarthritis and chronic pain.

Being overweight also negatively affects mental health and self-esteem. People with weight problems often experience social discrimination and ostracism, which leads to self-esteem issues, depression, and anxiety. Additionally, excess weight limits mobility and independence, limiting opportunities to participate in certain activities and affecting overall quality of life.

A holistic approach to weight loss fostering a healthy lifestyle is crucial to combat these adverse effects on well-being. This involves a combination of a balanced and varied diet, regular physical activity, and adequate stress management. It is essential to be accompanied by a professional health coach to obtain personalized advice and support in achieving your weight loss goals. Furthermore, developing a positive and self-compassionate mindset is crucial, remembering that well-being is not just a matter of weight but of overall balance between body and mind.

Remember, achieving a healthy lifestyle and losing weight takes time and effort, but the benefits to your wellness and health are invaluable. Take care of yourself and make conscious choices to live a life full of energy and vitality.

How to calculate Body Mass Index. BMI = kg/m2.

Divide your weight in kilograms by the square of your height in meters. Ex: 80kg: (1.70m x 1.70m)=47.05.

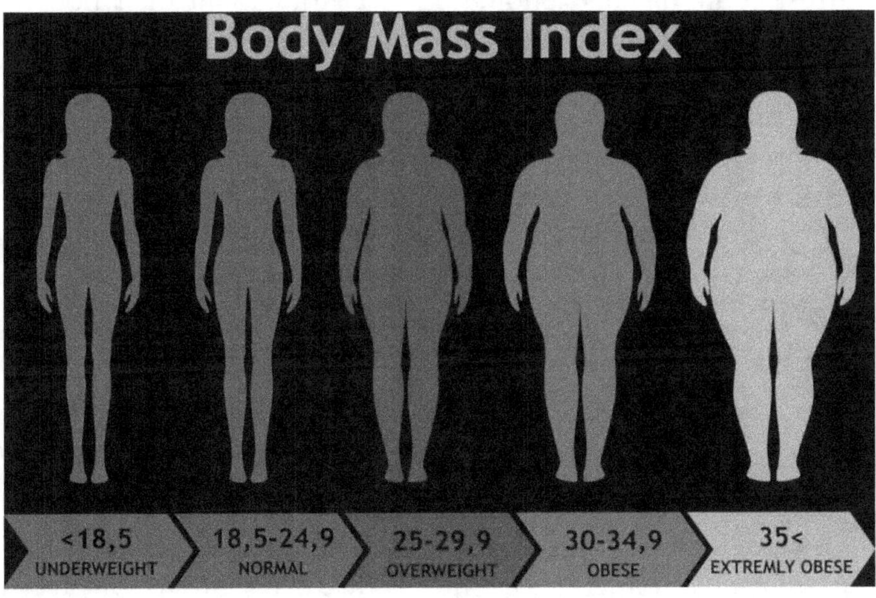

PREPARE FOR CHANGE

Accept your body

The path to healthy living and weight loss is complex and full of challenges. Often, those who are overweight experience frustration, dissatisfaction, and insecurity about their body. We address the topic of body acceptance, a fundamental aspect of embarking on a path of positive change.

Accepting your body does not mean giving up the desire to improve your health and lose weight, but instead embracing the knowledge that everybody is unique and deserves respect and care. The first step towards acceptance is to stop comparing yourself to the unrealistic beauty standards imposed by society and the media. Everybody has a different history and unique metabolism, so you must focus on your well-being rather than comparing yourself to others.

Another key to accepting your body is learning to talk to yourself kindly. Often, we rebuke ourselves for our physical appearance, creating a vicious cycle of insecurity and low self-esteem. Instead, learn to love and appreciate your body for what it is in this moment, recognizing that every progress you make toward a healthy lifestyle is cause for celebration.

Accepting your body is a process that takes time and patience. It would help if you remembered that losing weight and achieving a healthy life are not goals but the consequences of striking a balance between a complete diet and regular physical activity. Focus on small victories and daily progress; it will keep your attitude positive and motivated.

Finally, also remember that accepting your body, in addition to a gift you give to yourself, is also a positive example you give to others. By showing confidence and acceptance for your body, you inspire others to do the same.

In conclusion, accepting your body is fundamental to finding and implementing a healthy lifestyle and weight loss. Free yourself from adverse judgments, embrace love for yourself, recognize that everybody deserves respect and care, and prepare to embark on a positive and sustainable change path.

Your motivation

Motivation is critical to achieving any goal in life, including weight loss. When tackling overweight, motivation becomes even more crucial, as you often face challenges and obstacles that can cause you to give up.

The first thing to understand is that motivation must come from within you. You can't wait for someone else to push you to start this journey. You have to find that inner spark that pushes you to want to change and achieve better health and overall well-being.

One of the best sources of motivation is the image of yourself in the future. Visualize yourself as you would like to be, as you would like to feel. Imagine yourself with more energy, confidence, and satisfaction in life. This image will help you maintain focus and determination during your weight loss journey.

Another way to keep motivated is to set realistic and achievable goals. Especially in the beginning, setting small goals you can easily reach is essential. This will give you a sense of accomplishment and push you to keep moving forward.

Additionally, you must find a support system. Finding

someone or a group of people to share your journey with is extremely helpful. They will support you when you need encouragement and help you face your challenges.

Finally, remember to reward yourself. Give yourself a small reward whenever you reach a goal or overcome a challenge. This will give you a sense of gratification and motivation to continue your weight loss process.

Motivation for weight loss is a critical factor for success. Find what drives you internally, set realistic goals, seek support, and reward yourself. With strong motivation, you will overcome any challenge and achieve your weight loss goals without stress.

Create a supportive environment

Creating a supportive environment is critical in achieving a healthy lifestyle and losing weight without stress. Often, we are influenced by our surroundings more than we imagine. Therefore, it is vital to make conscious choices to make your environment an ally in your fight against being overweight.

Start with the kitchen, the heart of the home. This is where you make many of your food decisions. To create a supportive environment in the kitchen, start by eliminating high-calorie, unhealthy foods. Replace processed, high-sugar foods with healthier alternatives, such as fresh fruits, vegetables, lean proteins, whole grains, and supplementation. Organize your refrigerator and pantry to always have healthy foods on hand. Also, avoid shopping on an empty stomach and filling your cart with unnecessary foods.

In addition to cooking, the environment you live and work in significantly impacts your health and weight loss. Make your space comfortable and relaxing so you can reduce stress and anxiety, which often lead to poor food choices. Create a space dedicated to physical activity, such as a home gym or yoga room. Additionally, reduce exposure to tempting foods, such as sweets and unhealthy snacks, by keeping them out of sight and reach.

Finally, also involve the people around you in your healthy lifestyle goal. Share your intentions and ask for their support. Organize outdoor activities with friends and family, such as healthy walks or picnics. Together, you create a supportive environment that helps you achieve your goals in weight loss and healthy living.

Creating a supportive environment takes time, effort, and patience, but the results are excellent. Take control of your environment, and you will find yourself one step closer to achieving a healthy lifestyle and overcoming excess weight.

HEALTHY DIET

Importance of a balanced diet

The importance of a balanced diet cannot be stressed enough when it comes to achieving a healthy weight and maintaining a healthy lifestyle in the long term. For those who struggle with being overweight, a balanced diet becomes even more crucial to achieving the desired results without stress.

A balanced diet gives your body all the essential nutrients to function correctly. These nutrients include carbohydrates, proteins, healthy fats, vitamins and minerals. Adequate intake of each nutrient is critical to maintaining a healthy metabolic balance and promoting weight loss.

Regarding carbohydrates, choosing whole grains such as wholemeal bread, pasta, and wholegrain cereals is essential. These carbohydrates provide long-term energy and keep you feeling full for longer. At the same time, you must reduce your refined sugar and sweets intake, which can cause blood sugar spikes and lead to unwanted weight gain.

Protein is critical for building and repairing tissue and keeping muscles strong and healthy. Foods such as legumes, low-fat dairy products, eggs, fish, and lean meat are excellent sources of protein that can be integrated into your daily diet.

Healthy fats in olive and vegetable oils, nuts, and avocados are essential for the body to function correctly. These fats provide energy, help absorb fat-soluble vitamins, and promote satiety. However, it is necessary to consume them in moderation, as they are still sources of calories.

Finally, a balanced diet must include a variety of fruits and vegetables. These foods, rich in minerals, vitamins, and antioxidants, support overall health and help keep body weight under control.

Remember, a balanced diet is the key to achieving and maintaining a healthy weight and happy lifestyle in the long term. With the help of a professional wellness coach, you can create a personalized meal and fitness plan that fits your specific needs.

<h3 style="text-align:center">Conscious food choices</h3>

The food choices we make every day profoundly affect our health and body weight. For those who are overweight and want to adopt a healthy lifestyle and lose weight, it is essential to make informed food choices.

Awareness about the foods we put on our plates is the first step towards a healthier life. We must learn to read food labels and understand the ingredients and nutritional information. This will help us avoid foods high in saturated fats, added sugars, and sodium, often responsible for weight gain and related health problems.

Additionally, we must prioritize fresh, unprocessed foods. Lean proteins, whole grains, vegetables, fruits, and low-fat dairy products should be integral to our daily diet. These foods provide vital nutrients, vitamins, and minerals essential for our body without adding excess calories.

Another conscious food choice involves portion sizes. We often tend to eat more than necessary without realizing it. Learn to control the amount of food we put on our plates, avoiding overfilling it. You can use smaller plates and controlled portions to avoid overdoing calories and at the same time gradually reduce the size of your stomach.

Finally, it is important to remember to drink enough. Water is essential for the proper functioning of our body and can help control hunger and cravings for high-calorie foods. We should avoid carbonated, sugary, and alcoholic drinks, which are usually full of empty calories.

Making conscious food choices takes commitment and discipline but can affect our health and weight. Let's start today by making informed decisions about the foods we eat, transforming our lives towards a healthier lifestyle, and achieving our weight loss goals without stress.

Plan your meals

Meal planning is vital in achieving a healthy lifestyle and weight loss. Often, when we are overweight, we tend to eat in a disorganized and improvised way without considering the real needs of our bodies. However, with proper meal planning, we can achieve excellent results.

One of the initial steps in meal planning is establishing a weekly menu. This not only gives us a clear picture of our meals but also allows us to prepare in advance. Dedicate some time to create a well-balanced menu, incorporating various healthy, nutrient-rich foods. For a wholesome diet, remember to include fresh fruits and vegetables, lean proteins, whole grains, and healthy fats.

Once you have established your weekly menu, proceed with the shopping list. It will help you avoid purchasing impulses and maintain a healthier diet. Be sure to include all the ingredients needed to prepare your planned meals. Also, try to do your shopping after eating, so as not to be tempted by unhealthy foods.

When preparing meals, try to cook in larger quantities and save the extra portions for later meals. This will help you save time and avoid eating out or ordering ready-made foods. You can use plastic containers or bags to store food in the refrigerator or freezer.

In conclusion, meal planning is fundamental to healthy lifestyles and losing weight without stress. Create a weekly meal plan, a grocery list, and cook in advance. Remember to include healthy, nutritious foods and avoid impulse purchases. With proper planning, you will achieve your weight loss goals, maintain them, and enjoy a healthier, happier life.

Portions and calorie control

Many people who struggle with being overweight often wonder what the best way to control calories and manage portions is during their weight loss journey. The secret is finding a balance between what you eat and the amount of food you consume.

Portion control is essential to achieving and maintaining a healthy weight. Overweight people often eat more significant portions than necessary, mainly due to the size of the stomach, without realizing the excess calories they consume. It is crucial to learn to recognize the right quantities of food to drink and to satisfy your appetite without exceeding.

One way to control portions is to use smaller dinnerware, such as smaller plates and glasses. This psychological trick can help you feel full even with smaller amounts of food. Additionally, serving food in predefined portions is advisable rather than eating straight from the package or the serving dish. This allows you to have more precise control over the quantities and avoid finishing all the contents without realizing it.

In addition to portion control, paying attention to food calories is essential. Reading nutritional labels can be an excellent habit for understanding the calories in a food and making more informed choices. It is necessary to learn to recognize high-calorie foods and limit their consumption.

Another helpful tip is to pay attention to sugary drinks, which can contain many calories without providing a feeling of satiety. Choosing low-calorie beverages such as water, tea, or unsweetened coffee can help reduce your overall calorie intake.

Remember that portion and calorie control doesn't mean giving up the taste or satisfaction of food. Creating healthy and tasty dishes using fresh and nutrient-rich ingredients is possible without exceeding the quantities. Experiment with spices and seasonings to add flavor to your meals without increasing the calories.

In conclusion, portion and calorie control are critical elements in achieving a healthy lifestyle and weight loss success. Learning to manage the amount of food you consume and make conscious choices make a difference in reaching your health and wellness goals.

PHYSICAL ACTIVITY AND MOVEMENT

Benefits of physical exercise

Exercise is an essential element of healthy living and stress-free weight loss. Not only does it help you burn calories, but it offers a number of benefits for your body and mind. Let's explore the many benefits that regular physical activity offers to those who are overweight and want to adopt a healthier lifestyle.

One of the main benefits of exercise is weight loss. A minimal regular physical activity, combined with a balanced diet, helps burn excess calories and gradually achieve a healthy body weight. Furthermore, exercise helps tone muscles, making the body leaner and more defined.

In addition to weight loss, regular physical activity offers a number of other health benefits. Playing sports or doing aerobic activity, such as swimming or running, improves blood circulation, reduces blood pressure and increases cardiorespiratory resistance. This decreases the risk of heart disease, stroke and diabetes.

Exercise also positively impacts on your mental health. During physical activity, the body releases endorphins, chemicals that improve mood and reduce stress. Regular physical activity helps fight anxiety, depression and improve the quality of sleep.

Furthermore, exercise helps improve muscular endurance and strength, increasing energy and activity in everyday life. You feel stronger and more capable during your daily activities, such as play with your kids or climbing stairs or carrying groceries.

In conclusion, exercise is an essential element for achieving a healthy lifestyle and weight loss. In addition to helping you reduce body weight, a minimal regular physical activity provides many benefits for both your physical and mental health. So, begin now to take advantage of the benefits it offers to incorporate exercise into your daily routine, knowing your investing in your present and future health.

Recommended types of physical activity

Adding a pleasant physical activity to your daily routine is essential and within your reach, regardless of your current fitness level. This is key to maintaining a healthy life and losing weight without stress. Regular exercise helps burn calories and improves stamina, strength, and flexibility. Here are some types of physical activities that are accessible and recommended for those who are overweight and want to adopt a healthy lifestyle and lose weight.

1. Walk. Walking, as a physical activity, is accessible to anyone, and you can easily integrate it into your daily routine. Walking for at least 30 minutes daily helps burn calories, improve blood circulation, and reduce stress.

2. Swim. Swimming is a low-impact physical activity involving all the body's muscles. It is particularly suitable for those who are overweight, as the water supports the body weight, reducing joint stress.

3. Ride a bicycle. Cycling is an easy and fun way to burn calories and improve your fitness. You can cycle outdoors, enjoy nature, or use a stationary exercise bike at home.

4. Practice yoga. Yoga is a physical activity that combines fluid movements, conscious breathing, balance, and meditation. It is ideal for those who want to improve flexibility, reduce

stress, and tone muscles.

5. Train with weights. Weight training is excellent for building muscle and speeding up your metabolism. Start with light weights, or use your body resistance to start with push-ups and push-ups.

Consult with your family doctor and a certified fitness professional before embarking on any physical activity. Your doctor provides medical advice based on your health condition. At the same time, a fitness professional helps design a personalized exercise plan suiting your fitness level and goals. This step ensures that the activity is safe and tailored to your needs, giving you the confidence to start your fitness journey.

Remember, physical activity should be a way to care for your body and health, not a burden. Choose the exercises you enjoy most that fit into your lifestyle. This way, you'll find that losing weight and maintaining a healthy weight is achievable but also enjoyable and sustainable over time. Whether it's a leisurely walk in the park, a refreshing swim, or a challenging yoga session, find the activities that make you feel good and look forward to your next workout.

Create a workout routine

Those who struggle with being overweight feel overwhelmed when it comes to starting an exercise program. The fear of not being up to par or having enough time is a natural obstacle. However, creating a workout routine is easier than you think.

The first important step is to set realistic goals. Ask yourself what you want to achieve with your training. Do you want to lose weight? Do you want to improve your endurance? Or you want to feel more energetic and fit. You can plan your training when you are clear about your primary goal.

Regularity is essential to achieve lasting results. Dedicate at least three or four days a week to physical activity. Start with short training sessions, such as 30 minutes, and then gradually increase the time as you feel more comfortable.

Choose an activity that you enjoy and that suits your needs. Opt for a brisk walk, light jog, swimming, or aerobics class. The important thing is that you have fun and keep your motivation high in the long term.

Remember to also include resistance exercises in your training program. Weight training or using resistance bands helps you tone your muscles and burn more calories. Start with light weights and gradually increase the resistance as you feel stronger.

Finally, remember that training is not the only important factor in losing weight healthily. A balanced and complete diet and a healthy lifestyle are equally essential. Ensure you eat fruits, vegetables, lean proteins, and complex carbohydrates. Drink at least 2 liters of water and reduce, until eliminating, the consumption of processed and sugary foods.

Creating an exercise routine is a challenge. Still, you can achieve your weight loss goals and live a healthy lifestyle with determination and commitment. Remember to listen to your body and always make gradual progress. Good workout!

Overcome obstacles to exercise

Exercise is critical to achieving a healthy lifestyle and achieving desired weight loss. However, for many overweight people, it is difficult to overcome the obstacles that stand between them and regular physical activity. Let's explore helpful strategies to overcome these obstacles and make exercise sustainable.

One of the significant obstacles many people face is a need for more motivation. Often, the idea of starting an exercise program seems daunting and overwhelming. It's important to remember that exercise doesn't have to be intense or dull. Find an activity you love, like dancing, swimming, or taking a walk in nature. The important thing is to move and have fun doing it.

Another common obstacle is the need for more time. Our lives are busy, and finding time to exercise seems like a challenging task. However, there are many practical solutions you can take. For example, you can integrate physical activity into your daily routine by using the stairs or walking during lunch breaks and phone calls. Additionally, you can plan shorter but more intense training sessions, which require less time but still offer significant benefits.

Another common obstacle is a need for more social support. Having people who encourage and support you on your weight loss journey makes all the difference. Find one or more training partners or a support group to share your experiences and motivate each other. Also, involve your family and friends in making a lifestyle change so they can understand and support your choices.

Finally, remember to listen to your body. If you have pain or health problems, consult your doctor before starting any exercise program. Respect your body's limits to avoid injury and keep exercise enjoyable and safe.

Overcoming obstacles to exercise requires commitment and determination, but the results are worth it. Find the strategies that work best for you, and never give up. Remember, every small step towards a healthy lifestyle counts; it brings you closer to your weight loss and control goal.

MANAGE STRESS

Relationship between stress and overweight

Stress and being overweight are two problems that often go hand in hand in many people's lives. When under pressure, we tend to seek comfort in food, usually preferring fast and unhealthy options that lead us to gain weight. But what is the actual relationship between stress and overweight? How can we address both of these issues healthily and effectively?

Stress is our body's physiological response to a situation perceived as threatening or challenging. When stressed, our body produces cortisol, which influences our metabolism and nutrition. Some people eat more when stressed, often reaching for junk or comfort food to relieve emotional tension. This behavior leads to weight gain and a negative spiral of stress and overweight.

On the other hand, being overweight is also being a source of stress. People who struggle with their weight feel insecure and frustrated, and this increases their stress levels. Additionally, being overweight leads to health problems such as diabetes, hypertension, and cardiovascular disease, which further fuel stress.

To conquer this relationship between stress and overweight, adopting a healthy lifestyle and finding alternative ways to manage stress is essential. Doing physical activity helps reduce stress and maintain a healthy weight. Furthermore, following a balanced and nutritious diet is necessary, avoiding excesses of unhealthy food.

Therefore, stress management is also essential. Find relaxation techniques like yoga, meditation, or tai chi that help you reduce tension and improve overall well-being. Also, find enjoyable activities that distract you from the temptation to compulsive eating when you're under stress.

In conclusion, the relationship between stress and overweight is complex but manageable. By adopting a healthy lifestyle, combining physical activity, stress management techniques, and a balanced diet, you can address these problems effectively. Remember that physically and emotionally caring for yourself is essential for healthy living and stress-free weight loss.

Stress management techniques

Stress is a factor that often contributes to weight gain and maintaining an unhealthy lifestyle. For this reason, learning to manage stress is essential if you want to lose weight and live healthily.

Several stress management techniques help reduce anxiety and daily tension. One of the most effective is the practice of meditation. Meditation allows you to focus on the present, relax, and let go of negative thoughts. Find a quiet time and place every day to meditate; it will benefit your mind and body significantly.

Another helpful technique is regular exercise. Physical activity helps burn calories and lose weight and positively affects stress. During training, the body releases endorphins, chemicals that improve mood and reduce stress. Choose a physical activity you enjoy and dedicate time to it daily. It is an effective way to manage stress and promote weight loss.

Deep breathing is another simple and effective technique for reducing stress. Breathe deeply and slowly. It helps you relax your body and calm your mind. When you feel stressed, you tend to breathe shallowly. Take a few minutes and focus on your breathing. It makes a big difference.

Finally, remember the importance of rest and quality sleep. Lack of sleep increases stress levels and negatively affects weight loss. Make sure you get enough sleep and adopt a regular sleep routine. It promotes a calmer mind and a healthier body.

Learning to manage stress is an essential step to achieve a healthy lifestyle and lose weight in a lasting way. Try these techniques and adapt them to your needs, and you will immediately notice the difference in the path to a more balanced and happy life.

Strategies to avoid emotional overeating

Emotional binge eating, or the habit of eating to compensate for negative emotions, is a common challenge for many people trying to achieve healthy living and weight loss. Recognizing and addressing this behavior is critical to achieving lasting success in reaching your weight goals.

Here are some practical strategies to avoid emotional binge eating:

1. Practice mindfulness. Take the time to reflect on what you're feeling before reaching for the food. Ask yourself if you're starving or trying to satisfy an emotional need.

2. Find healthy alternatives. Instead of turning to food for comfort, try exploring other activities that help you manage stress or negative emotions. Take a walk, listen to relaxing music, keep a diary of your feelings, or drink 2 glasses of water.

3. Create an emotional care routine. Set aside time daily to care for yourself in general. It helps you reduce any emotional overeating. Find activities that relax and make you feel good, such as taking a warm bath, massaging yourself with body lotion, reading a book, or practicing yoga.

4. Identify your emotional buttons. Pay attention to situations or events that trigger emotional binge eating. It could

be stress at work, an argument with your partner, or boredom. Once identified, think of healthy ways to deal with them without resorting to food and apply them.

5. Seek support. Talk to a trusted friend or seek professional help. It is extremely helpful in managing emotional binge eating. Share your experiences and receive support. It makes you feel less lonely and more determined to achieve your goals.

Remember, emotional binge eating is a common challenge. Still, with the proper awareness and strategies, you avoid turning to food to deal with your emotions. Be kind to yourself and take care of your emotional well-being as you work towards your ideal weight and a healthier life.

KEEP MOTIVATION

Celebrate successes

One of the fundamental keys to achieving a healthy lifestyle and weight loss is learning to celebrate successes along the way. We often focus only on the end goals and neglect the small milestones we achieve. But it is important to remember that every step forward is a reason to celebrate and feel pride in the goal achieved.

When you begin a health and weight loss journey, it's common to have some ups and downs. There are moments in which you feel entirely motivated and full of energy. In contrast, in other moments, you fall prey to demotivation or think of giving up. It is precisely in these moments that celebrating successes becomes even more critical.

But what exactly does it mean to celebrate successes? It can be as simple as a small gesture to reward progress made. For example, you could treat yourself to a beauty treatment, a relaxing massage, or buy an item you like. The important thing is to recognize your commitment and dedicate time all to yourself.

Plus, sharing your successes with others is an excellent source of motivation. Talk to friends and family about what you have achieved and be encouraged by their support. You can also look for an online community or support group that shares your goals. Together, you can celebrate successes and overcome challenges.

Finally, remember to celebrate successes on an internal level, too. Every time you reach a goal or overcome a challenge, take a moment to appreciate your hard work and determination. Remember that you are on the right path and that every success brings you closer to your goals.

Celebrating successes is a powerful tool for maintaining motivation and enthusiasm on your journey to a healthy lifestyle and weight loss. Please don't neglect the small milestones; celebrate them and enjoy the process. Your health and well-being deserve to be celebrated!

Deal with the fallout

You will inevitably encounter setbacks in losing weight and a healthy lifestyle. It is essential to understand that relapses are part of the process and should not be a reason for discouragement or demotivation. Approach them with the right mindset. It is essential for maintaining motivation and achieving your goals.

When overweight, it is expected to fall into temptation and give in to old unhealthy eating habits. This happens to every person, even those who have adopted a healthy lifestyle for some time. Remember that a relapse doesn't mean failure but simply a step back on the road to wellness.

It is helpful to follow some practical advice to deal with relapses effectively. First, it's important not to get caught up in guilt or the feeling of having ruined everything. Accept the relapse as part of the journey and own your actions. It is the starting point for regaining control.

Another fundamental tip is to analyze the causes that led to the relapse. Identify triggers, such as stress or negative emotions. It helps you better understand your eating behaviors and make necessary changes.

Once you understand the causes, focus on the goal and resume the path toward a healthy lifestyle. Resume good eating habits and regular physical activity. This is the key to overcoming relapses and returning to the right path.

Finally, you must have social support. Sharing your experiences with people in the same situation as you is a great help. Find a support group or friend with whom you can share your successes and difficulties. It will provide you with the encouragement you need to overcome relapses.

Dealing with relapses is integral to a healthy lifestyle and weight loss. Accept them, analyze them, and overcome them with determination and support. Here are the basic steps to achieve your goals. Remember that every small step forward is a success and that although there will be obstacles, nothing can stop your determination to live a healthy and happy life.

Involve friends and family

When you embark on a weight loss and healthy lifestyle journey, involving friends and family makes all the difference. In fact, having a solid and encouraging support system makes the weight loss journey more enjoyable and rewarding.

First, it's essential that you clearly communicate to your loved ones your goal to lose weight and adopt a healthier lifestyle. Express your intentions openly and sincerely. It will help you get the support you need. Tell them your choice to change is about you and your desire to live a healthier, happier life together.

Involving friends and family in your exercise routine is a fun way to spend time together and reach your goals simultaneously. Organize group walks, runs, or training sessions. Involve your loved ones in outdoor activities such as walking, Nordic, trekking, or cycling. Remember that the important thing is to have fun together and find ways to stay active.

Likewise, involving your family in preparing healthy meals is the best opportunity to experiment with new recipes and create a healthy eating environment. Ask your loved ones to participate in choosing ingredients and preparing meals. By doing this, you promote more nutritious food choices for everyone.

Finally, remember to celebrate your successes together with your friends and family. Share your progress and accomplishments, encouraging each other along the way. Organize a dinner where you cook healthy and tasty dishes and celebrate when you reach intermediate goals. Surrounding yourself with people who support and encourage you will make your weight loss journey more rewarding.

Remember that involving friends and family in your weight loss journey makes the process more enjoyable and sustainable. Be bold, ask for help, and affect the people you care about. Manifest your weight loss goals and enjoy a proud, healthier life.

Continue to commit to healthy living

Maintaining a healthy lifestyle after reaching your goal is a challenge. It requires consistency and dedication, especially for those who struggle with being overweight. However, despite the difficulties, you can achieve your goal of losing weight and living healthy.

The first step towards a healthy life is personal commitment. Decide to make a change and, with determination, follow a regular exercise routine and a balanced diet. Don't be discouraged by occasional failures; find the motivation to keep working towards your goal.

Another key to success is finding the perfect weight loss program, a combination that fits your lifestyle and needs. Consult professionals in the sector and together create a personalized plan for you. Remember that every person is different, and what works for some may not work for you. Be inclined to try new strategies and adapt your weight loss program based on your results.

Additionally, experiment with different types of physical

activity to find the one you like best. You don't need to join the gym if you don't like the environment; taking long walks in the open air or practicing a sport you are passionate about is sufficient. Maintaining consistent physical activity to burn calories and improve overall fitness is essential.

Finally, remember the importance of a positive mental state. The path to weight loss is treacherous and full of obstacles. Keep an open and confident mind. Seek support from friends and family, participate in support groups, and work with those who can help you stay motivated and overcome challenges.

Remember, weight loss, maintaining the result, and a healthy lifestyle is a long-term journey. Keep working towards your goals and celebrate every little success along the way. Your determination and perseverance will eventually lead you to your ideal weight and enjoy a healthy and fulfilling life.

ADDRESS MYTHS AND UNREALISTIC EXPECTATIONS

Debunks weight loss myths

Weight loss is a much-discussed topic often surrounded by myths and false beliefs. It is essential to clarify these misunderstandings to follow a healthy and effective weight loss path. Let's reveal some of the most widespread myths about weight loss and see practical tips to achieve your goals without stress.

Myth 1: Skipping meals makes you lose weight faster.

The reality is that skipping meals leads to a decrease in metabolism and an increased feeling of hunger, making you compensate with an unhealthy snack. Instead, following a balanced diet and consuming frequent but controlled meals to keep the metabolism active is essential.

Myth 2: Cutting out carbs helps you lose weight.

Carbohydrates should not be demonized. They are an essential source of energy for your body. Choosing wholemeal carbohydrates such as wholemeal bread, pasta, and cereals is necessary, avoiding refined ones. It is also essential to control portions to avoid excess calories.

Myth 3: Miracle supplements make you lose weight quickly.

There are no magic weight loss supplements. They should always be added to a balanced diet and regular exercise. If you feel the need to supplement your diet, consult those who are competent in the matter to obtain personalized advice.

Myth 4: Exhausting physical activity is the only way to lose weight.

Physical activity is a component of weight loss, but you can do it without overdoing it. Dedicate 30 minutes daily to moderate physical activity such as brisk walking, swimming, or cycling. The important thing is to be constant over time.

Debunking these myths will help you get on a healthier, more sustainable weight loss journey. Always listen to your body, be patient, and don't look for miracle solutions. You will achieve your goals without stress with a balanced diet, adequate supplementation, regular exercise, and a positive attitude.

Create realistic and sustainable goals

Setting realistic and sustainable goals is crucial when it comes to losing weight. We often want to achieve immediate and drastic results, but this approach is counterproductive in the long term. It is imperative to take a gradual and sustainable approach to achieve lasting weight loss and maintain a healthy lifestyle.

First, setting realistic goals is essential. This means avoiding setting unattainable or impractical goals. For example, if you want to lose 10 kilos in a week, it is unrealistic and also dangerous for your health. Please understand that healthy weight loss happens gradually and that you must give your body time to adapt.

Another important aspect is the sustainability of the objectives. There's little point in losing weight quickly if you regain it soon after. You must adopt a sustainable weight-loss approach to avoid the so-called yo-yo effect. This means focusing on healthy, lasting eating habits rather than drastic, temporary diets.

One way to create realistic and sustainable goals is to break the journey into a series of minor stages. For example, if you intend to lose 40 pounds, focus on losing 4-6 pounds per month, about 3.5 oz daily. This makes the goal psychologically more manageable and allows you to maintain motivation over time. improve

Additionally, remember that weight loss isn't just about the numbers on the scale. Also, focus on enhancing your overall health and achieving a healthy lifestyle. This includes increasing physical activity, which increases muscle mass, adopting a balanced diet, and managing stress positively.

In conclusion, creating realistic and sustainable goals is essential for lasting weight loss and a healthy lifestyle. Avoid drastic approaches and focus on small changes you can maintain over time. Remember, weight loss is a long-term commitment. It requires patience and consistency.

Accept that every path is unique

On the path to healthy living and weight loss, accepting that every journey is unique is critical. Each individual has their own characteristics, goals, and challenges to face. There is no magic formula that works the same for everyone. It is essential to understand that what works for one person may not work for another.

We often let ourselves be influenced too much by other people's success stories, thinking that by following the same path, we will achieve the same results. The truth is that everybody is different and responds differently to certain stimuli and strategies. What works for you may not work for me, and vice versa.

Accepting that every path is unique also means accepting yourself as you are and accepting your body. Don't constantly compare yourself only with others, but focus on yourself and your needs. Learn to listen to your body and adapt your weight loss strategies based on its responses.

This means being open-minded to different possibilities and approaches to help you achieve your goals. Experiment, try new strategies, and find what works best for you.

Accepting that every path is unique frees you from the stress and pressure of following the same rules as everyone else. It allows you to be kinder to yourself and appreciate every little progress you make. Remember that life is a journey and that every step you take towards a healthy life is a success worth celebrating.

So, accept that every path is unique and embrace your journey towards a healthy life and weight loss without stress, aware that you are on the right path, even if it seems different from that of others, always with the support of a professional of the sector.

KEEP YOUR RESULTS

Strategies to maintain your weight achieved

Have you finally reached your ideal weight and now wonder how to maintain it over time? Don't worry; here are some effective strategies to maintain weight and live a healthy life without stress.

The first fundamental strategy is to adopt a balanced and sustainable lifestyle. Continue to eat healthy and balanced by choosing fresh, nutrient-rich foods and avoiding processed foods and foods rich in added sugars. Remember that the secret is balance and moderation.

Another essential strategy is to maintain constant physical activity. Regular exercise always helps you burn calories and improve your overall health. Stick with the activity you enjoy, whether walking, running, swimming, or yoga, and keep doing it at least 3-4 times a week. Keep your body active.

Another crucial aspect of maintaining your weight is continuing to manage stress. Continue to apply your relaxing and managing stress methods, such as meditation, yoga, or simply taking time for what you love. Now that you have learned to recognize stress, deal with it immediately, healthily, and positively.

Also, remember the importance of social support. Keep

active involvement with family and friends on your weight maintenance journey. Share with them your successes and challenges overcome to keep your motivation high and the encouragement necessary to persevere until you have finally adopted the new eating habit and the new healthy lifestyle.

Finally, remember to supplement if you feel you cannot give your body all the nutrients it needs through nutrition.

Maintaining your weight is a long-term commitment and requires perseverance and determination. Still, with these simple and right strategies and a balanced approach, you can enjoy a healthy life and maintain your ideal weight with joy.

Maintain a healthy lifestyle forever

For many people, maintaining a healthy lifestyle seems like an impossible challenge. The numerous temptations surrounding us and daily commitments often appear as obstacles holding us back from caring for ourselves. However, our determination to make changes guides us to reach and maintain our ideal weight and a balanced lifestyle.

The first attitude to maintaining a healthy lifestyle for the long term is to adopt a positive mindset. Accept that the path to health requires commitment and consistency. This is critical. Small steps make a difference, so keep your spirits up if results are not coming immediately.

One of the keys to maintaining a healthy lifestyle is nutrition. Choose nutritious foods and avoid those rich in saturated fats and sugars. It is essential. Opt for a balanced, nutritious diet rich in fruit, vegetables, whole grains, and lean proteins. It helps you reach and maintain your ideal weight.

Additionally, regular exercise is another vital part of maintaining a healthy lifestyle. Find a physical activity that you enjoy, and that fits your lifestyle. As mentioned, it could be a daily walk, a yoga session, or a gym membership. The important thing is that you move and do at least 30 minutes of physical activity a day.

Remember the importance of rest and stress control. Sleep enough and find healthy ways to manage tension. As mentioned, meditation, free time dedicated to your favorite hobbies, and socializing contribute to maintaining your healthy lifestyle forever.

Finally, remember to supplement if your diet needs to be nutritionally complete or sufficiently suited to your lifestyle. Integration is the contemporary magic formula that makes up for the lack of nutrients in industrial foods, the lack of time to shop and cook, and imagination in the kitchen.

Finally, give space to water. Remember, 2 liters between meals is the minimum necessary to activate your metabolism.

The path to a healthy lifestyle is more of a marathon than a race. Be patient if old habits sometimes come back, smile, and carry on. Enjoy every little success along the way, and never give up. With determination and consistent effort, you will reach your weight goals. Meanwhile, you will acquire new eating and lifestyle habits. You will, therefore, be able to maintain the best version of yourself forever, comfortably and peacefully.

Have a good trip.

Andrea.

CONCLUSIONS

Summary of the main points covered

Let's revisit these essential points, which are theoretical and practical steps to intelligently and stress-free achieve your weight loss and healthy lifestyle attitudes and maintain them forever.

We looked at the importance of proper nutrition. How to create a balanced diet rich in essential nutrients such as lean proteins, fruits, vegetables, and whole grains. How can we choose fresh foods and limit the consumption of processed foods to eliminate them eventually? Essential for maintaining a healthy weight.

We looked at the importance of physical activity. How do you find the exercise that best suits your needs and integrate it into your daily routine? How to burn calories and tone your body, from aerobics to weight lifting.

We discussed the importance of rest and quality sleep. How sleep habits affect your metabolism and overall well-being. How to improve your sleep quality and create a relaxation routine before bed. How to create a comfortable environment in your bedroom.

We've delved into maintaining a positive and motivated mindset during your weight loss journey. These strategies will help you face obstacles, overcome temptations, and be kind to yourself along the way. Remember, weight loss is a gradual process, but with these tools, you can supplement your diet, be accompanied by professionals, and stay on track.

Trusting that this information is helpful to you, I wish you success in implementing the best version of yourself with joy, lightness, and lots of energy!

BIBLIOGRAPHY

Scarsi, Andrea 2024. Stop Dreaming: Accept Yourself As You Are.

Scarsi, Andrea 2020. Happy To Be Happy: The Grand Manual Of Happiness.

Scarsi, Andrea 2012. The Secret of Meditation: The Inner Dimension.

Scarsi, Andrea 2015 The Art of Worrying: How To Enter And Exit It At Will.

ABOUT THE AUTHOR

Andrea Scarsi is a master of meditation who defines himself as a mystic, metaphysician, author, musician, and holistic coach when he uses his works to share a dimension of being, lifestyle, and knowledge founded on communion with the absolute.

Born in Venice, Italy, in 1955, he began practicing yoga and spiritism and experimenting with telepathy at fifteen. Following a near-death experience, he contacted alien and transdimensional entities at eighteen. At twenty-four, on his first trip to India, he found himself a vegetarian and in the world of meditation led by India and the Spiritual Master Osho. He received Swami Prem Sandesh as a new name, which he wears in specific environments.

He has often traveled, especially to India, residing for long periods in Nepal, the Philippines, Brazil, and Buddhist Southeast Asia: Japan, Thailand, Sri Lanka, Hong Kong, Laos, China, and Tibet. He has explored local places and cultures, met people, and participated in ritual and religious practices.

Over time, he delved into various meditative techniques for awakening consciousness, energy rebalancing, and personal evolution, which he practices and teaches. He studied philosophy and earned a Doctorate in Metaphysical Science and various diplomas, such as Holistic Life Coach, Reiki Grand Master, Master of Crystals, Shamanism, Meditation and Massage, and Wellness Coach. He's also into cellular nutrition and Network Marketing.

In 1991, he married Krisana, and they now live in Venice, Italy. You can reach him at andrea.scarsi@yahoo.com and https://www.youtube.com/@ScarsiAndrea.

BOOKS BY ANDREA SCARSI

Answers For The Soul: Fragments of Eternal Wisdom
Blessings! Dedicated to Osho
Extraterrestrial Channeling: Alien Abduction Syndrome
Happy To Be Happy: The Grand Manual Of Happiness
Home Sweet Home Staging: Easy Is Right
How To Ask A Woman Out: Gentlemen Only
Indigo Crystal Rainbow and Diamond: Tell Themselves
Journey To The Underworld: First Level Shamanic Procedures Manual
Make Your Own Vineyard: Ex Vite Vita
O Iguana! My Iguana! Herbivore is Beautiful
Pearls of Wisdom: Tales of Ordinary Metaphysics
Reiki First Degree Manual
Reiki Second Degree Manual
Reiki Third Degree Manual
Romance Ain't Love Pollution: Romance Will Never Die
Seeds Of Enlightenment: The Buddha Within
Stop Dreaming! Accept Yourself As You Are
Tarot Reading Essentials: The New Basic Meaning Manual
The Art of Persuasion: How to Achieve Your Goals Ethically
The Art of Worrying: How to Enter and Exit it at Will
The Master And The Assassin: An Ordinary Zen Story
The Secret Of Meditation: The Inner Dimension
The Secret Of Metaphysical Science: Our Eternal Journey Through Infinite
The Silence of The Absolute: Satsang with Sandesh
Vegetarian Cuisine: Reasons Objections Recipes
Walking The Dogs: A Dialogue A Manual
Zen The Sense Of Nonsense: Anecdotes For Synaptic Deprogramming

MANTRA BY ANDREA SCARSI (SANDESH)

Mantras Maha Mantras
The Mantra Experiment
The Mantra Way
Om Namo Supernova
Amāvasya
Lingamananda

A mantra is a Verbal Being acting as a bridge between the human and the divine. It carries our prayer, thankfulness, and gratitude. It is an entity in its own right. When we recite or sing it to communicate with the superior dimension, in addition to words and sound, we also employ intention, energy, devotion, and focus. All this raises us immediately. It increases our emotional state and makes us touch God.

A mantra is an introspective event turning to the multiple aspects of the One by evoking its symbolic names: Shiva, Brahma, Vishnu, Ganesha, Laxmi, Saraswati, Gurudev, and Shanti, names representing the infinite manifestation of the cosmic cycle. They are magic formulas for amending the universal present, resolving the apparent fragmentation, and recreating the union of consciousness with what is.

A mantra is to be recited and sung without interruption to convey the intact message, and breathing comes between recitations. Let's get lost in the mantra and let the vehicle, the human, and the divine become one. That's the power of the mantra. We recite it and go deeper until melting what we were before, our intention, recitation, sound, and collective energy, and manifesting unity once again, the yoga of consciousness, the absolute presence, whose supreme name is Om.

BOOKS BY ANDREA SCARSI IN ITALIAN

21 Giorni: Diario di un Ritiro Spirituale

A Proposito di Osho: Conferenze di Un Suo Discepolo

Basta Sognare: Accettati Come Sei

Benedizioni!: Dedicato a Osho

Benvenuti ad Atlantide: Cristalli e Chakra Riequilibrio di Primo Livello

Breve Storia Dei Sogni: Nella Visione Occidentale

Canalizzazioni Extraterrestri: Sindrome da Rapimento Alieno

Casa Dolce Casa Vendesi: Home Staging Facile

Come Ripristino Le Capacità Del Mio Cervello

Dhyana Yoga: Unione Con L'Essenza

Dispense Reiki Primo Livello

Dispense Reiki Secondo Livello

Dispense Reiki Terzo Livello Master

Felici Di Essere Felici: Il Grande Manuale Della Felicità

Guarire il Sé Ombra: Aneddoti Di Alleggerimento Di Carico

Il Lato Positronico: Ridondanze Di Un Androide

Il Maestro e l'Assassino: Una Consueta Storia Zen

Il Segreto della Meditazione: La Dimensione Interiore

Il Segreto della Scienza Metafisica: Il Nostro Eterno Viaggio nell'Infinito

Il Silenzio dell'Assoluto: Satsang con Sandesh

Immagina: E Accelera la Tua Crescita Personale

Indaco Cristallo Arcobaleno e Diamante: Si Raccontano

La Cucina Vegetariana: Motivazioni Obiezioni Ricette

L'Arte della Persuasione: Come Raggiungere Eticamente i Propri Obiettivi

L'Arte della Preoccupazione: Come Entrarci e Uscirne a Piacere

L'Arte di Cambiare: Modella la Tua Vita

L'Arte di Invitare una Donna: Solo per Gentiluomini

Le Compatibilità Zodiacali: Trova l'Anima Gemella con l'Astrologia

Lettura dei Tarocchi: Manuale dei Significati di Base

Massaggio Olistico: Manuale delle Procedure di Base

Menando Il Can Per L'Aia: Un Dialogo Un Manuale

Notiziario Reiki: Delle Attività Mensili Svolte

Perle di Saggezza: Racconti di Ordinaria Metafisica

Risposte per l'Anima: Frammenti di Eterna Saggezza

Semi di Illuminazione: Il Buddha Interiore

Sovrappeso? No Problem! Consigli per Una Vita Sana e Perdita di Peso Senza Stress

Transizione Vegetariana: Per la Pecora che si Crede Leone

Viaggio nel Mondo di Sotto: Manuale di Procedura Sciamanica di Primo Livello

Zen Il Senso del Non Senso: Aneddoti di Deprogrammazione Sinaptica

Thank you for reading
Overweight? No Problem!
Andrea Scarsi

www.ingramcontent.com/pod-product-compliance
Lightning Source LLC
Chambersburg PA
CBHW051706250726
48653CB00007B/2886